APPROPRIATING YOUR HEALING

Amb Promise Ogbonna

CONTENTS

WHY I WROTE THIS BOOK!

I am sent to Publish All the Words of God's Heavenly Kingdom Life for the Restoration of all.

I am not writing human philosophy. I am not writing as a hobby neither am I writing to entertain but to bring Spiritual light, impart, Spiritual, Wisdom and Power to build your faith and transform your life! I have a Mandate from The Lord Jesus Christ to write and these Words are published to meet man's needs in every area of life! This Book, therefore, is published in obedience to the Command of the Lord to make His Words of Life and Wisdom, Solutions and Power available to address every aspect of human needs.

I can say as Paul wrote "My message and my preaching were not in the persuasive language of philosophy, but in demonstration of the Spirit and of power; in order that your faith should rest, not on human philosophy, but on the power of God." 1Corinthians 2:4-5 (BBE)

"For the Kingdom of God is based, not on words, but on power." 1Corinthians 4:20 (BBE)

The Life Publishing Mandate

The Lord sent me to Publish All The Words of His Heavenly Kingdom Life for ALL mankind!

Jesus' last words is to Preach and Publish the Goodnews with proofs to every creature and among all nations (Mark 13:10; 16:15; Matthew 24:14).

The Lord gave us the Goodnews to publish and spread among all nations (Psalm 68:11; Mark 13:10).

In the Book of Esther, the enemy wrote and spread the words of death worldwide to destroy God's people and souls that God loves. [See Esther 3].

But at the command of the king, a new decree and words of life were written and spread to reach everyone (every creature) everywhere that the first words of death had reached. [See Esther 8].

This is our task. We have been given the New Covenant, Heavenly Kingdom, Words of Life to publish and spread to reach every creature everywhere worldwide. The Goodnews is that no one needs to die again! The old decree has been changed. Everyone can now live and enjoy peace and prosperity where each lives. That is why Ontop Mission Life Publishers Company. We are Publishing, Spreading and Bringing the Gospel of Christ and All the Words of life to every creature everywhere.

I will like to share some of the encounters with the Lord Jesus Christ that gave birth to The Life Publishing Mandate and why this Book and my other books:

1. On 2-5-95, Jesus Christ and I stood on the balcony of a great beautiful mansion in Heaven whose foundation I couldn't see (see Amos 9:6). He showed me Preachers, driven by selfishness and being used by the enemy, walking on people's heads and shoulders as their platform to preach. The people were hungry, thirsty, weeping, trampled upon and yet yearning for the TRUTH (see Amos 8:11-13). I saw My Lord shaking His head in disgust. He also brought to my view those in hell and I saw their agony and pain and what a sight it was! Afterward, as we beheld the abuse of His people, He pointed His right hand towards them and said to me, "See what is happening to the people I died for. "The Lord Jesus gave me A WELL USED COPY OF THE BIBLE and said to me "GO and tell them (The Preachers and The People) to Repent and Believe The Gospel Only and they will be Restored." I asked 'How

will I do it? And He said to me, "BE SEPARATE! Go, I send YOU as My Ambassador and Witness with My Authority and Power: Publish The Word, Stop anything after their destruction, Raise, Build and Plant them as My Ambassadors. Let them know the truth. Teach All The TRUTH and Spread them as My Seed ALL over the earth and restore all things."

2. On 6-7-96, The Lord Jesus Christ came to me again and said, "It is well" and gave me a copy of THE BIBLE and said to me, "Take: This is My Staff of Office" – My Authority and Power. After The LORD gave me His Staff of Office [The Word], I saw something like a mist or cloud appear out of the Word and as I watched, a horse emerged from 'within the mist' and jumped about and stopped. The Lord told me The Word is creative and created the horse and is My Rod for working Miracles, Wonders and Signs. I am to Go with it to all, as Moses went with his ROD, and "Stop anything after man's destruction, Bring Healing, Liberty and Restoration to all; Raise, Build and Plant Christ's Ambassadors everywhere and Restore all things."

3. On 20-5-97, I was given a BIBLE and 2 BIROS by Arch. Benson A. Idahosa in a conference that took place in a place like a stadium. And he said to me, "Go and Proclaim and Publish The Everlasting Gospel of Jesus Christ worldwide and deliver the full benefits to all. This Gospel of The Kingdom must be preached in all the world for a witness unto all nations!

4. On 18-11-03, The Lord spoke to me again ON WRITING, and said to me "Write all the hidden mysteries I show you and I will ensure it gets to all the Nations. Prophetic writings is what unveils, reveals, makes known the revelation of the mystery hidden for ages long past. The surest way of unveiling the Gospel and proclaiming Jesus Christ the Lord, is through prophetic writings as God commanded so that all nations will believe and obey God.

5. On 26-11-03, The Lord spoke to me saying, "Write what people can read and understand. It's most important. Your writing must be readable and understandable. Write in such a way that a primary school pupil can read and understand My Words. "The common people heard me gladly." Everyone must read and

understand My Words that you write.

6. On 2-10-04, The Lord Jesus explained to me the vision of 2one fifths s /95 where I Stood with Him on the Balcony of the Mansion in Heaven and He showed me Preachers using the shoulders and heads of people as their platform to preach. They were hungry, thirsty and trampled underfoot yet yearning for the reality. And The Lord commanded me to WRITE and publish His Words for the downtrodden and for all."

7. On10-12-04, The Lord said to me "Write in a book all the Words that I have spoken to you" and He gave me Jeremiah 30:2.

8. On 04-04-05, The Lord said to me "Publish the Word and bring healing, liberty and restoration to all everywhere." See Psalm 68:11 and Psalm 107:20.

9. On 23-12-05, The Lord said to me: Publish The Words, Publish The Works, Publish The Wonders, Make My Deeds Known, and Let Everyone See My Glory Everywhere.

10. On 01-03-13, The Holy Ghost said to me:
Publish the Works of Jesus Christ everywhere
Advertise the Doings of Jesus Christ the Lord.
Make known the Miracles of Jesus Christ the Lord.
Bind the Testimony of the Acts of the Lord Jesus Christ's
Be My Witness of all My Signs and Wonders everywhere.
Share Testimonies of All I AM Doing forever.

Go and Tell All everywhere of All My Miracles and Wonders and Signs and All I have done and commanded you.

The Lord said to me "All who believe that I sent you and receive you as My Ambassador and receive your Words as My Words will experience all the Father sent me to make available to humanity!"

Like Peter, I can tell you "We have not followed cunningly devised fables, when we made known unto you the power and coming of our Lord Jesus Christ, but were eyewitnesses of his majesty." 2Peter 1:16

Beloved, every Word written in this Book is from The Lord and are His Wisdom and Heaven's Solutions packaged and released to deal with your challenges, solve your problems and meet your needs.

Read with an open heart, Believe and Receive The Truth and Pick the Lessons and engage them.

I know you will experience The One who is The Author, Perfecter and Finisher of your faith and Who is The Real Author of this Book. He is Jesus Christ, The Son of The Living God. And He is the Same yesterday and today and forever!

"O LORD, how manifold are Your works! In wisdom You have made them all. The earth is full of Your possessions." Psalm 104:24

I guarantee you that you will never be the same again as you embrace God's Wisdom in This Book!

God Bless you.

Your brother and His Steward for the benefit of all,

Ambassador Promise Ogbonna

THE HEAVENLY MANDATE & VISION

The Heavenly Mandate

To Preach The Everlasting Gospel to Everyone everywhere, Stop anything after man's destruction, Bring Healing, Liberty and Restoration to ALL; Raise, Build and Plant All as Christ's Ambassadors on His Living Mission everywhere and Restore all things!

The Heavenly Vision

To Restore All Things Everywhere at All Cost and By All Means! Acts 3:21

FIRST WORDS

To be Healed, you do nothing!

That's an unusual and a very strange statement to make yet it is so very true.

You are not to labour to be Healed You are not to wear yourself out in search of healing or spend fortunes to secure healing. You merely receive what belongs to you and has been fully paid for.

God says "Himself [Jesus Christ] bore our sins in His own body on the tree, that we, having died to sins, might live for righteousness--by whose stripes you were healed." 1 Peter 2:24

Notice what God says: By whose stripes you were healed! If 'YOU were healed' then 'YOU are healed'!

"He [Jesus Christ] Himself took our infirmities [or diseases] and bore our sicknesses." Matthew 8:17

Notice again what God who cannot lie says about you: Himself [Jesus Christ] TOOK YOUR diseases and BORE [carried away] YOUR sicknesses. What Jesus Christ took and carried away and destroyed on the TREE where He was crucified and declared IT IS FINISHED stands finished forever! That settles the problem of sickness and disease forever for all who will believe! All you need to do is to believe and receive!

Jesus Christ speaking in John 3:14-17 says "And as Moses lifted up the serpent in the wilderness, even so must the Son of man be lifted up: That whosoever believeth in him should not perish, but have eternal life. For God so loved the world, that he gave his only begotten Son, that whosoever believeth in him should not perish, but have everlasting life. For God sent not his Son into the world to condemn the world; but that the world through him might be saved [healed, delivered, made whole, restored to sound health and preserved]."

Notice that every single person that was bitten by the serpent in Numbers 21:4-9 that LOOKED on God's provision by faith, LIVED! They didn't do anything to be healed. They only looked and got healed. Whatever was the distance between where they were and where the serpent of brass made by Moses at God's command was placed was immaterial. All that looked by faith got healed instantly and lived. That's how simple healing is for all who will believe in God's Provision today! God never made healing difficult, only religion does.

The Lord God wants all the sick to be healed by faith. LOOK and be healed of any and every sickness.

Healing has never been made simpler! Look up by faith and see Jesus on the Cross and be healed and live.

This Book is on a Divine Assignment and Mission: To Bring to YOU all The Living Word made flesh brought to the people of God in His days on earth. Read with an open heart. Its YOUR season of Restoration to God's Divine Health Plan. You shall not die sick but be healed and live. And all you need is Faith!

CHAPTER 1

APPROPRIATING YOUR HEALING

To be Healed, you do nothing!

That's an unusual and very strange statement to make yet it is so very true.

To be Healed, you do nothing! You merely receive what belongs to you and has been fully paid for.

"Who Himself bore our sins in His own body on the tree, that we, having died to sins, might live for righteousness--by whose stripes you were healed." 1Peter 2:24

"He Himself took our infirmities and bore our sicknesses." Matthew 8:

Jesus Christ speaking in John 3:14-16 says "And as Moses lifted up the serpent in the wilderness, even so must the Son of man be lifted up: That whosoever believeth in him should not perish, but have eternal life. For God so loved the world, that he gave his only begotten Son, that whosoever believeth in him should not perish, but have everlasting life."

To have a good understanding of the above passage, let us read the passage that Jesus referred to.

Numbers 21:4-9

4 "And they journeyed from mount Hor by the way of the Red sea, to compass the land of Edom: and the soul of the people was much discouraged because of the way.

5 And the people spake against God, and against Moses, wherefore have ye brought us up out of Egypt to die in the wilderness? for there is no bread, neither is there any water; and our soul loathes this light bread.

6 And the LORD sent fiery serpents among the people, and they bit the people; and much people of Israel died.

7 Therefore the people came to Moses, and said, we have sinned, for we have spoken against the LORD, and against thee; pray unto the LORD, that he take away the serpents from us. And Moses prayed for the people.

8 And the LORD said unto Moses, make thee a fiery serpent, and set it upon a pole: and it shall come to pass, that every one that is bitten, when he looks upon it, shall live.

9 And Moses made a serpent of brass, and put it upon a pole, and it came to pass, that if a serpent had bitten any man, when he beheld the serpent of brass, he lived."

Notice that every single person that was bitten by the serpent that LOOKED, LIVED. They didn't do nothing to be healed. Whatever was the distance between where they were and where the serpent of brass made by Moses at God's command was immaterial. All that looked got healed instantly and lived.

That is how The Lord wants all the sick to be healed. LOOK and be healed of any and every sickness.

Healing has never been made simpler! Look and be healed and live.

To Secure your Healing and Live in Health, you Do Something.

Proverbs 4:20-22

20 "My son, attend to my words; incline thine ear unto my sayings.

21 Let them not depart from thine eyes; keep them in the midst of thine heart.

22 For they are life unto those that find them, and health to all their flesh."

The word of God is medicine and you must take responsibility of taking it. Not only must you hear it, you must speak or confess it with your mouth to write it in your heart and keep it there.

"Write them [The Word of God] upon the table of thine heart:" Proverbs 3:3

How do you write the Word in your heart? By speaking the Word with your mouth.

"My heart is inditing a good matter: I speak of the things which I have made touching the king: my tongue is the pen of a ready writer." Psalm 45:1

"My son, keep my words, and lay up my commandments with thee. Keep my commandments, and live; and my law as the apple of thine eye. Bind them upon thy fingers, write them upon the table of thine heart." Proverbs 7:1-3

The Word is a seed and must be planted into the soil of your heart for it to produce.

In Mark 5:25-30 and Luke 8:41-43, the woman with the issue of blood secured her healing of a plague that had lasted for 12 years by speaking or sowing the seed into her heart.

"Now a certain woman had a flow of blood for twelve years, and had suffered many things from many physicians. She had spent all that she had and was no better, but rather grew worse. When she heard about Jesus, she came behind Him in the crowd and touched His garment. For she said, "If only I may touch His clothes, I shall be made well." Immediately the fountain of her blood was dried up, and she felt in her body that she was healed of the affliction. And Jesus, immediately knowing in Himself that power had gone out of Him, turned around in the crowd and said, "Who touched My clothes?" But His disciples said to Him, "You see the multitude thronging You, and You say, 'Who touched Me?'" And He looked around to see her who had done this thing. But the woman, fearing and trembling, knowing what had happened to her, came and fell down before Him and told Him the whole truth. And He said to her, "Daughter, your faith has made you well. Go in peace, and be healed of your affliction." Mark 5:25-34

"So it was, when Jesus returned, that the multitude welcomed Him, for they were all waiting for Him. And behold, there came a man named Jairus, and he was a ruler of the synagogue. And he fell down at Jesus' feet and begged Him to come to his house, for he had an only daughter about twelve years of age, and she was dying. But as He went, the multitudes thronged Him. Now a woman, having a flow of blood for twelve years, who had spent all her livelihood on physicians and could not be healed by any, came from behind and touched the border of His garment. And immediately her flow of blood stopped. And Jesus said, "Who touched Me?" When all denied it, Peter and those with him said, "Master, the multitudes throng and press You, and You say, 'Who touched Me?'" But Jesus said, "Somebody touched Me, for I perceived power going out from Me." Now when the woman saw that she was not hidden, she came trembling; and falling down before Him, she declared to Him in the presence of all the people the reason she had touched Him and how she was healed immediately. And He said to her, "Daughter, be of good cheer; your faith has made you well. Go in peace." Luke 8:41-48

Sow the seed.

Luke 8:11 says "Now the parable is this: The seed is the word of God."

"Another parable put he forth unto them, saying, The kingdom of heaven is like to a grain of mustard seed, which a man took, and sowed in his field: Which indeed is the least of all seeds: but when it is grown, it is the greatest among herbs, and becometh a tree, so that the birds of the air come and lodge in the branches thereof. Another parable spake he unto them; The kingdom of heaven is like unto leaven, which a woman took, and hid in three measures of meal, till the whole was leavened." Matthew 13:31-33

Why sow the seed? "For the seed shall be prosperous; the vine shall give her fruit, and the ground shall give her increase, and the heavens shall give their dew; and I will cause the remnant of this people to possess all these things." Zechariah 8:12

"He himself bore our sins in his body on the tree, that we might die to sin and live to righteousness. By his wounds you have been healed." 1 Peter 2:24 (RSV)

"This was to fulfil what was spoken by the prophet Isaiah, "He took our infirmities and bore our diseases." Matthew 8:17 (RSV)

Everything is in the past Tense. He accomplished All, Receive faith.

"And as Moses lifted up the serpent in the wilderness, so must the Son of man be lifted up, that whoever believes in him may have eternal life." For God so loved the world that he gave his only Son, that whoever believes in him should not perish but have eternal life." John 3:14-16; Numbers 21:4-9

God does not want to heal you. God has healed you already. Jesus Christ does not want to heal you. He has done everything to be done for you to be healed. Jesus said "It is finished!"

All that needed to be done for you to be healed has been done completely. It is now over to you. It is your Faith and obedience to The Word of God that you need to appropriate your healing.

God does not want to Heal you. He has healed you. And God wants you to spend all your days in Health.

Healing is an accomplished work ahead. You only need to Receive by faith so that you can experience and enjoy your healing if you are still sick.

Psalms 103:3

"Who forgives all thine iniquities; who heals all thy diseases;"
Salvation/Healing is already accomplished.

John 3:14-16

14 "And as Moses lifted up the serpent in the wilderness, even so must the Son of man be lifted up:

15 That whosoever believeth in him should not perish, but have eternal life.

16 For God so loved the world, that he gave his only begotten Son, that whosoever believeth in him should not perish, but have everlasting life."

(Numbers 21:4-9)- The way to receive Healing. But if you must enjoy Health, then you have a responsibility.

3John 2

"Beloved, I wish above all things that thou mayest prosper and be in health, even as thy soul prospereth." Soul Prosperity, Prosperity and Health.

Proverbs 3:1-2,5-10

1 "My son, forget not my law; but let thine heart keep my com-

mandments:

2 For length of days, and long life, and peace, shall they add to thee.

5 Trust in the LORD with all thine heart; and lean not unto thine own understanding.

6 In all thy ways acknowledge him, and he shall direct thy paths.

7 Be not wise in thine own eyes: fear the LORD, and depart from evil.

8 It shall be health to thy navel, and marrow to thy bones.

9 Honour the LORD with thy substance, and with the firstfruits of all thine increase:

10 So shall thy barns be filled with plenty, and thy presses shall burst out with new wine."- Wealth.

Proverbs 4:1-2,10,13,20-22

1 "Hear, ye children, the instruction of a father, and attend to know understanding.

2 For I give you good doctrine, forsake ye not my law.

10 Hear, O my son, and receive my sayings; and the years of thy life shall be many.

13 Take fast hold of instruction; let her not go: keep her; for she is thy life.

20 My son, attend to my words; incline thine ear unto my sayings.

21 Let them not depart from thine eyes; keep them in the midst of thine heart.

22 For they are life unto those that find them, and health to all their flesh." Health.

Exodus 15:26

"And said, If thou wilt diligently hearken to the voice of the LORD thy God, and wilt do that which is right in his sight, and wilt give ear to his commandments, and keep all his statutes, I will put none of these diseases upon thee, which I have brought upon the Egyptians: for I am the LORD that heals thee."

Hebrews 13:8

"Jesus Christ the same yesterday, and today, and forever."

John 10:10

"The thief cometh not, but for to steal, and to kill, and to destroy: I am come that they might have life, and that they might have it more abundantly" Life/Health/Abundance.

How to Maintain Prosperity/Health.

Luke 8:11

"Now the parable is this: The seed is the word of God."

Zechariah 8:12

"For the seed shall be prosperous; the vine shall give her fruit, and the ground shall give her increase, and the heavens shall give their dew; and I will cause the remnant of this people to possess all these things."

Keep Sowing The Seed for Health and Wealth.

God has healed you already. But God wants you to enjoy Divine Health.

Mankind's healing is God's entire responsibility (Receive by faith).

The Believer's Health is His Responsibility- (obey The Living Word).

To Receive by faith, you do nothing. To Have by obedience, you Do something-obey.

CHAPTER 2

WHY GOD WILL HEAL AND
BLESS A SINNER AND

What to Do After Receiving Your Healing and Blessing. God will HEAL or BLEESS the worst sinner if only he/she believes. Faith is the only Reason why God will do anything for anyone.

Mark 9:23

"Jesus said unto him, if thou canst believe, all things are possible to him that believeth."

Christ healed the Syrophoenician woman's daughter because of her faith. (Mark 7:24-30).

Christ healed the woman with the issue of blood because of her faith. (Mark 5:24-34).

Christ healed the Centurion's servant because of his great faith. (Matthew 8:5-13; Luke 7:1-10).

Lack of faith will hinder people from receiving their healing and blessings-Matthew 13:58; Mark 6:5-6.

God reckoned Abraham's faith for Righteousness. (Romans 4:9B).

We preach the Word of faith (Romans 10:6-8,17). For a detailed account, read Romans 10:6-18.

The word of faith has all it takes to accomplish all God desires upon the earth today.

Abraham was not born again when God called him. He only believed the word of God and his faith in God compelled God to input His own righteousness upon Abraham and also bless him. Why did God do so?

He did so to show us Gentiles that if only we can believe God's word, all the word is sent to do or accomplish in our lives will become realities.

Faith moves God's hand to release whatever we believe him for. It is the word that builds faith into the lives (heart) of the unbelievers and imparts same into them. And once they can receive the word into their heart and believe it, whatsoever they heard, received and believed the word for must be done. (Romans 10:9-10; Proverbs 4:1-2,20-22; Mark 9:23; Habakkuk 2:4).

After you have believed and Received God's word into your heart, what do you do?

1. Confess the word of life only.

Proverbs 4:20-23

20 "My son, attend to my words; incline thine ear unto my sayings.

21 Let them not depart from thine eyes; keep them in the midst of thine heart.

22 For they are life unto those that find them, and health to all their flesh. 23 Keep thy heart with all diligence; for out of it are the issues of life."

Romans 10:9-10

9 "That if thou shalt confess with thy mouth the Lord Jesus, and shalt believe in thine heart that God hath raised him from the dead, thou shalt be saved.

10 For with the heart man believeth unto righteousness; and with the mouth confession is made unto salvation."

Proverbs 18:20-21

20 "A man's belly shall be satisfied with the fruit of his mouth; and with the increase of his lips shall he be filled.

21 Death and life are in the power of the tongue: and they that love it shall eat the fruit thereof."

Isaiah 57:19

"I create the fruit of the lips; Peace, peace to him that is far off, and to him that is near, saith the LORD; and I will heal him."

Proverbs 15:4A

"A wholesome tongue is a tree of life:"

2. Keep away from all evil communications/communicators.

2Corinthians 6:14

"Be ye not unequally yoked together with unbelievers: for what fellowship hath righteousness with unrighteousness? and what communion hath light with darkness?"

1Corinthians 15:33

"Be not deceived: evil communications corrupt good manners."

Psalms 1:1

"Blessed is the man that walketh not in the counsel of the ungodly, nor standeth in the way of sinners, nor sitteth in the seat of the scornful."

Ephesians 4:29

"Let no corrupt communication proceed out of your mouth, but that which is good to the use of edifying, that it may minister grace unto the hearers."

Colossians 3:8

"But now ye also put off all these; anger, wrath, malice, blasphemy, filthy communication out of your mouth."

3. Always be in the midst of believers.

Proverbs 27:17

"Iron sharpens iron; so, a man sharpens the countenance of his friend."

Hebrews 10:25

"Not forsaking the assembling of ourselves together, as the manner of some is; but exhorting one another: and so much the more, as ye see the day approaching."

Psalms 133:1-3

1 "Behold, how good and how pleasant it is for brethren to dwell together in unity!

2 It is like the precious ointment upon the head, that ran down upon the beard, even Aaron's beard: that went down to the skirts

of his garments;

3 As the dew of Hermon, and as the dew that descended upon the mountains of Zion: for there the LORD commanded the blessing, even life for evermore."

Luke 5:17

"And it came to pass on a certain day, as he was teaching, that there were Pharisees and doctors of the law sitting by, which were come out of every town of Galilee, and Judaea, and Jerusalem: and the power of the Lord was present to heal them."

Acts 2:42-47

42 "And they continued steadfastly in the apostles' doctrine and fellowship, and in breaking of bread, and in prayers.

43 And fear came upon every soul: and many wonders and signs were done by the apostles.

44 And all that believed were together, and had all things common;

45 And sold their possessions and goods, and parted them to all men, as every man had need.

46 And they, continuing daily with one accord in the temple, and breaking bread from house to house, did eat their meat with gladness and singleness of heart,

47 Praising God, and having favour with all the people. And the Lord added to the church daily such as should be saved."

Acts 4:30-37

30 "By stretching forth thine hand to heal; and that signs and wonders may be done by the name of thy holy child Jesus.

31 And when they had prayed, the place was shaken where they were assembled together; and they were all filled with the Holy Ghost, and they spake the word of God with boldness.

32 And the multitude of them that believed were of one heart and of one soul: neither said any of them that ought of the things which he possessed was his own; but they had all things common.

33 And with great power gave the apostles witness of the resurrection of the Lord Jesus: and great grace was upon them all.

34 Neither was there any among them that lacked: for as many as were possessors of lands or houses sold them, and brought the

prices of the things that were sold,

35 And laid them down at the apostles' feet: and distribution was made unto every man according as he had need.

36 And Joses, who by the apostles was surnamed Barnabas, (which is, being interpreted, The son of consolation,) a Levite, and of the country of Cyprus,

37 Having land, sold it, and brought the money, and laid it at the apostles' feet."

Acts 5:12-16

12 "And by the hands of the apostles were many signs and wonders wrought among the people; (and they were all with one accord in Solomon's porch.

13 And of the rest durst no man join himself to them: but the people magnified them.

14 And believers were the more added to the Lord, multitudes both of men and women.)

15 Insomuch that they brought forth the sick into the streets, and laid them on beds and couches, that at the least the shadow of Peter passing by might overshadow some of them.

16 There came also a multitude out of the cities round about unto Jerusalem, bringing sick folks, and them which were vexed with unclean spirits: and they were healed everyone."

1 Corinthians 5:4

"In the name of our Lord Jesus Christ, when ye are gathered together, and my spirit, with the power of our Lord Jesus Christ,"

Hebrews 12:18-24

18 "For ye are not come unto the mount that might be touched, and that burned with fire, nor unto blackness, and darkness, and tempest,

19 And the sound of a trumpet, and the voice of words; which voice they that heard intreated that the word should not be spoken to them any more:

20 (For they could not endure that which was commanded, and if so, much as a beast touch the mountain, it shall be stoned, or thrust through with a dart:

21 And so terrible was the sight, that Moses said, I exceedingly

fear and quake:)

22 But ye are come unto mount Sion, and unto the city of the living God, the heavenly Jerusalem, and to an innumerable company of angels,

23 To the general assembly and church of the firstborn, which are written in heaven, and to God the Judge of all, and to the spirits of just men made perfect,

24 And to Jesus the mediator of the new covenant, and to the blood of sprinkling, that speaks better things than that of Abel."

Matthew 18:16-20

16 "But if he will not hear thee, then take with thee one or two more, that in the mouth of two or three witnesses every word may be established.

17 And if he shall neglect to hear them, tell it unto the church: but if he neglects to hear the church, let him be unto thee as a heathen man and a publican.

18 Verily I say unto you, Whatsoever ye shall bind on earth shall be bound in heaven: and whatsoever ye shall loose on earth shall be loosed in heaven.

19 Again I say unto you, that if two of you shall agree on earth as touching anything that they shall ask, it shall be done for them of my Father which is in heaven.

20 For where two or three are gathered together in my name, there am I in the midst of them."

4. Abound Steadfast, unmovable.

1Cornthiasn 15:58

"Therefore, my beloved brethren, be ye steadfast, unmovable, always abounding in the work of the Lord, forasmuch as ye know that your labour is not in vain in the Lord."

5. Always have a great expectation.

Proverbs 23:18

"For surely there is an end; and thine expectation shall not be cut off."

Psalms 37:37

"Mark the perfect man, and behold the upright: for the end of that man is peace."

6. Stand Having Done All.

Ephesians 6:13-14

13 "Wherefore take unto you the whole armour of God, that ye may be able to withstand in the evil day, and having done all, to stand.

14 Stand therefore, having your loins girt about with truth, and having on the breastplate of righteousness;"

7. Rejoice and Give God thanks always.

Hebrews 13:15

"By him therefore let us offer the sacrifice of praise to God continually, that is, the fruit of our lips giving thanks to his name."

Psalms 50:5,14-15

5 "Gather my saints together unto me; those that have made a covenant with me by sacrifice.

14 Offer unto God thanksgiving; and pay thy vows unto the most High:

15 And call upon me in the day of trouble: I will deliver thee, and thou shalt glorify me."

1 Thesalonians 5:18

"In everything give thanks: for this is the will of God in Christ Jesus concerning you."

Note: You must always avoid wrong conversations- Psalms 1:1; 1 Corinthians 15:33.

CHAPTER 3

HEALING- FREEDOM FROM THE HOUSE OF BONDAGE

Exodus 13:14

"And it shall be when thy son asks thee in time to come, saying, what is this? that thou shalt say unto him, by strength of hand the LORD brought us out from Egypt, from the house of bondage:"

Acts 10:38

"How God anointed Jesus of Nazareth with the Holy Ghost and with power: who went about doing good, and healing all that were oppressed of the devil; for God was with him."

Luke 4:18-19

18 "The Spirit of the Lord is upon me, because he hath anointed me to preach the gospel to the poor; he hath sent me to heal the brokenhearted, to preach deliverance to the captives, and recovering of sight to the blind, to set at liberty them that are bruised,

19 To preach the acceptable year of the Lord."

Luke 13:16

"And ought not this woman, being a daughter of Abraham, whom Satan hath bound, lo, these eighteen years, be loosed from this bond on the sabbath day?"

Sickness is imprisonment. It is slavery. It means enslavement.

It is confinement in the house of bondage. It is to live under oppression. It is being under the custody of the oppressor. Sickness is satanic rule over a life in the house of bondage.

That precious soul, a daughter of Abraham, a daughter of the covenant was confined to satanic chain of bondage with sickness. She was bound. But Christ the Lord gave her freedom.

The Lord of the liberation mandate did not abandon her in Satan's house of bondage. Jesus loosed her and set her free from her bondage. Jesus healed her. Healing is freedom from the house of bondage-sickness and oppression of the devil.

Exodus 13:14 says, "And it shall be when thy son asks thee in time to come, saying, what is this? That thou shalt say unto him, BY STRENGHT OF HAND (SHEER POWER) THE LORD BROUGHT US OUT FROM EGYPT, FROM THE HOUSE OF BONDAGE" (God's sheer power- The Living Word and The Holy Spirit- Isaiah 11:1-2).

Psalms 103:3 & 107:20 – He forgave them all their sins; he HEALED all their sickness. It was by sending His word through Moses that deliverance/salvation was enforced via The Living Word He sent and the signs and wonders he performed through His servant.

But He went in and through Moses. The Living word and The Rod of God were God's means of showing His Sheer Strength and power.

Psalms 105:37

"He brought them forth also with silver and gold: and there was not one feeble person among their tribes."

He brought them forth (Psalms 107:20; 103:3-Salvation/deliverance/healing) also with silver and gold and there was not one feeble person among their tribes. (See 3John 2). All were healed and delivered out of their destructions (Psalms 107:11,17-20).

It was the Lord (The Lord that heals thee (Exodus 15:26) that brought them out of the house of slavery/bondage/sickness. (Exodus 13:14; Luke 13:16; Acts 10:38).

The Lord is called "The I am that I am" (Exodus 3:14).

The Lord that changes not. (Malachi 3:6).

The same Yesterday, and Today and Forever. (Hebrews 13:8).

He is our healer today as He has always been. (Isaiah 53:4-5; 1Peter 2:24; Matthew 8:17; Acts 10:38; Malachi 3:6; Exodus 3:14; Hebrews 13:8). So, You Cannot Die in Bondage.

CHAPTER 4

2 Chronicles 30:18-20

18 "For a multitude of the people, even many of Ephraim, and Manasseh, Issachar, and Zebulun, had not cleansed themselves, yet did they eat the Passover otherwise than it was written. But Hezekiah prayed for them, saying, the good LORD pardon every one

19 That prepares his heart to seek God, the LORD God of his fathers, though he be not cleansed according to the purification of the sanctuary.

20 And the LORD hearkened to Hezekiah, and healed the people."

Hezekiah prayed and God healed them. God's forgiveness of his people was only expressed by their healing.

Genesis 20:17

"So, Abraham prayed unto God: and God healed Abimelech, and his wife, and his maidservants; and they bare children."

2 Chronicles 7:14

"If my people, which are called by my name, shall humble themselves, and pray, and seek my face, and turn from their wicked ways; then will I hear from heaven, and will forgive their sin, and will heal their land."

Exodus 15:26

"And said, If thou wilt diligently hearken to the voice of the LORD thy God, and wilt do that which is right in his sight, and wilt give ear to his commandments, and keep all his statutes, I will put none of these diseases upon thee, which I have brought upon the Egyptians: for I am the LORD that heals thee."

Healing is for the forgiven and obedient one.

Exodus 23:25-26

25 "And ye shall serve the LORD your God, and he shall bless thy bread, and thy water; and I will take sickness away from the midst of thee.

26 There shall nothing cast their young, nor be barren, in thy land: the number of thy days I will fulfil."

Healing for the obedient.

Psalms 103:3

"Who forgives all thine iniquities; who heals all thy diseases;"

Forgiveness/Healing.

Matthew 9:2-6

2 "And, behold, they brought to him a man sick of the palsy, lying on a bed: and Jesus seeing their faith said unto the sick of the palsy; Son, be of good cheer; thy sins be forgiven thee.

3 And, behold, certain of the scribes said within themselves, this man blasphemes.

4 And Jesus knowing their thoughts said, wherefore think ye evil in your hearts?

5 For whether is easier, to say, thy sins be forgiven thee; or to say, Arise, and walk?

6 But that ye may know that the Son of man hath power on earth to forgive sins, (then saith he to the sick of the palsy,) Arise, take up thy bed, and go unto thine house."

Healed and forgiven.

John 20:21-23

21 "Then said Jesus to them again, Peace be unto you: as my Father hath sent me, even so send I you.

22 And when he had said this, he breathed on them, and saith unto them, Receive ye the Holy Ghost:

23 Whose so ever sins ye remit, they are remitted unto them; and whose so ever sins ye retain, they are retained."

Healing.

Mark 16:15-18

15 "And he said unto them, Go ye into all the world, and preach the gospel to every creature.

16 He that believeth and is baptized shall be saved; but he that believeth not shall be damned.

17 And these signs shall follow them that believe; In my name shall they cast out devils; they shall speak with new tongues;

18 They shall take up serpents; and if they drink any deadly thing, it shall not hurt them; they shall lay hands on the sick, and they shall recover."

Healing.

1Peter 2:24

"Who his own self bare our sins in his own body on the tree, that we, being dead to sins, should live unto righteousness: by whose stripes ye were healed."

Jesus died for our healing/forgiveness.

Isaiah 53:3-4

4 "Surely he hath borne our griefs, and carried our sorrows: yet we did esteem him stricken, smitten of God, and afflicted.

5 But he was wounded for our transgressions, he was bruised for our iniquities: the chastisement of our peace was upon him; and with his stripes we are healed."

Jesus died for our healing/forgiveness.

Matthew 8:17

"That it might be fulfilled which was spoken by Esaias the prophet, saying, Himself took our infirmities, and bare our sicknesses."

Jesus died for our healing/forgiveness.

Psalms 107:20

"He sent his word, and healed them, and delivered them from their destructions."

God sent His word to heal to show His forgiveness.

Proverbs 13:17

"A wicked messenger falls into mischief: but a faithful ambassador is health."

Ambassadors are healers.

John 17:18

"As thou hast sent me into the world, even so have I also sent them into the world."

Ambassadors are healers.

Please Note: TO SURRENDER ONES LIFE MEANS We Becomes His Ambassadors.

What was Jesus Focus?

1John 3:8

"He that commits sin is of the devil; for the devil sinneth from the beginning. For this purpose, the Son of God was manifested, that he might destroy the works of the devil."

Destroy the works of the devil.

Acts 10:38

"How God anointed Jesus of Nazareth with the Holy Ghost and with power: who went about doing good, and healing all that were oppressed of the devil; for God was with him."

Heal all the oppressed.

Luke 13:16

"And ought not this woman, being a daughter of Abraham, whom Satan hath bound, lo, these eighteen years, be loosed from this bond on the sabbath day?"

Loose the bound from bondage.

Luke 4:18-19

18 "The Spirit of the Lord is upon me, because he hath anointed me to preach the gospel to the poor; he hath sent me to heal the brokenhearted, to preach deliverance to the captives, and recovering of sight to the blind, to set at liberty them that are bruised,

19 To preach the acceptable year of the Lord."

Preach Prosperity to the poor, (cloth the naked, feed the hungry, House the houseless, preach the good news to the poor).

-Proclaim Release to the captives.

-Set at liberty the oppressed.

-Preach the era of Jubilee for all enslaved ones.

To be His Ambassador means we;

-Become Shepherd for the homeless.

-Advocates for the poor.

- Proclaim of human rights.

-Creators of new liberating structures.

-We become His healers and perform the above roles as Jesus did.

Note: Something in man perishes if he is not able to find and do the work connected with his deepest beings, but if he does not do the work at all, the very self is lost.

1.Moses came a leader of the Revolution in his time and pharaoh commanded his death and destruction.

2.Jesus came a leader of the Revolution in His time and Herod/Pilate commanded his death and destruction.

Anytime Revolution leaders are born, the kingdom of evil is threatened/shaking and will be out to kill the leader. But just as they weren't able to stop God before, they cannot stop His purposes/intentions today, so they kill them "because they are the seeds from which the subversives shall grow (Lamentation 3:36-37).

CHAPTER 5

HEALING AND LISTENING

There Is no Important Service in all the world than LISTEN-ING.

The sick cannot be healed until they are LISTENED TO.

And Christ's Ambassadors cannot be healers until they know how to LISTEN.

LISTENING breeds healing, provokes Healing and Enforces Healing. LISTEN and HEAL AND BE Healed.

Listening does not only have to do with standing/sitting or being with the sick to hear them or talk to them. You can hear by Reading (Romans 10:17), and you speak to by writing/publishing Living Books inspired by The Holy Spirit and sending them to the sick. (See Psalms 68:11; 107:20; Romans 10:14-15).

Books /Publications bridge the gap between the hearers and the speakers.

- Read and You will hear/listen to the pain of the sick.

- Then speak/write/publish and send The Living Word and you'll be talking to the sick and bringing about their healing.

This is God's method. God listens while in heaven to the pains of the sick in all earth. Then God packages the word and sends it to all the sick in the earth. Those who read/believe/receive God's sent word are healed and delivered from their destructions.

None sick can be healed until he/she is listened to and none can be a healer until such knows how to listen.

It is as we listen first that solutions to HEALING are delivered/communicated, believed and received and experienced.

Hear This:

THINK AND LIVE.

THINK AND BE FREE.

THINK AND BE HEALED.

LONG TIME FOR BROODING MARKS A LIFE FREE OF PHARAOH'S RULE- SLAVERY/WORK/BONDAGE. (See Exodus 5:10-14).

Meditation/Brooding is the key to the cure/healing of all forms of enslavements. (Proverbs 23:7; Joshua 1:8; Psalms 1:2-3).

Freedom from bondage is rooted in thinking. If you can think, any form of slavery, regardless of how long it has been will come to an end.

Moses thought and the result was the termination of 430yrs slavery. Think and be free.

CHAPTER 6

HEALTH RESORATION FOR ALL

I saiah 42:21-22 (KJV)

21 "The LORD is well pleased for his righteousness' sake; he will magnify the law, and make it honourable.

22 But this is a people robbed and spoiled; they are all of them snared in holes, and they are hid in prison houses: they are for a prey, and none delivereth; for a spoil, and none saith, Restore."(Romans 8:19-23; Acts 10:38; Luke 4:18-19; Psalms 107:10-22; Psalms 68:11).

Jeremiah 30:11-17 (KJV)

11 "For I am with thee, saith the LORD, to save thee: though I make a full end of all nations whither I have scattered thee, yet will I not make a full end of thee: but I will correct thee in measure, and will not leave thee altogether unpunished.

12 For thus saith the LORD, thy bruise is incurable, and thy wound is grievous.

13 There is none to plead thy cause, that thou mayest be bound up: thou hast no healing medicines.

14 All thy lovers have forgotten thee; they seek thee not; for I have wounded thee with the wound of an enemy, with the chastisement of a cruel one, for the multitude of thine iniquity; because thy sins were increased.

15 Why cries thou for thine affliction? thy sorrow is incurable

for the multitude of thine iniquity: because thy sins were increased, I have done these things unto thee.

16 Therefore all they that devour thee shall be devoured; and all thine adversaries, every one of them, shall go into captivity; and they that spoil thee shall be a spoil, and all that prey upon thee will I give for a prey.

17 FOR I WILL RESTORE HEALTH UNTO THEE, AND I WILL HEAL THEE OF THY WOUNDS, SAITH THE LORD; because they called thee an Outcast, saying, this is Zion, whom no man seeks after."

If someone can cry Restore, then He will act.

Acts 3:21

"Whom the heaven must receive until the times of restitution of all things, which God hath spoken by the mouth of all his holy prophets since the world began."

Jesus will wait until all in any form of bondage (Romans 8:19-23) are restored.

We (Calmers/Life-rep) are sent here to Restore all –Emancipation and Recover all things.

We are to bring His health to all (Proverbs 13:7).

We must Restore health to the sick: that's why we are here.

God is committed to Restoring health unto all and healing all that are oppressed by the devil of all their sickness, disease and wounds.

CHAPTER 7

You need a good sleep to maintain a sound healthy body. Lack of proper sleep is a major reason why so many cannot enjoy sound health even after they have been healed. Cares, worries, anxieties, fretting, fears, all contribute to why many find it difficult to sleep at night.

So much money is wasted/spent on drugs to buy sleep. The best beds, under the best roofs, in the best quarters, under the best security devices cannot give or cause you to sleep.

And if you cannot sleep soundly, even if you sleep for 2-4hours daily, you'll have strong challenges with your health.

God prepared sleep for man to enhance healing, Health and longevity. Therefore, whatever can take sleep away from you (robs you of sleep) is ultimately going to rob you of life (health/longevity).

What has Our Loving Father Done Concerning our Sleep?

Psalms 127:2

"It is vain for you to rise up early, to sit up late, to eat the bread of sorrows: for so he giveth his beloved sleep."

God giveth His beloved sleep.

Psalms 3:5-6

5 "I laid me down and slept; I awaked; for the LORD sustained me.

6 I will not be afraid of ten thousands of people, that have set themselves against me round about."

Psalms 4:8

"I will both lay me down in peace, and sleep: for thou, LORD, only makest me dwell in safety." (Job 11:18-19)

1Samuel 26:12

"So, David took the spear and the cruse of water from Saul's bolster; and they get them away, and no man saw it, nor knew it, neither awaked: for they were all asleep; because a deep sleep from the LORD was fallen upon them."

Psalms 139:7-10,17-18

7 "Whither shall I go from thy spirit? or whither shall I flee from thy presence?

8 If I ascend up into heaven, thou art there: if I make my bed in hell, behold, thou art there.

9 If I take the wings of the morning, and dwell in the uttermost parts of the sea;

10 Even there shall thy hand lead me, and thy right hand shall hold me.

7 How precious also are thy thoughts unto me, O God! how great is the sum of them!

18 If I should count them, they are more in number than the sand: when I awake, I am still with thee."

Proverbs 3:24

"When thou lie down, thou shalt not be afraid: yea, thou shalt lie down, and thy sleep shall be sweet."

Leviticus 26:6

"And I will give peace in the land, and ye shall lie down, and none shall make you afraid: and I will rid evil beasts out of the land, neither shall the sword go through your land."

Psalms 17:15

"As for me, I will behold thy face in righteousness: I shall be satisfied, when I awake, with thy likeness."

He recreates, remolds/works on you while you sleep-between 12.00 and 3.00am and you get up renewed and in his likeness.

Jeremiah 31:26

"Upon this I awaked, and beheld; and my sleep was sweet unto me."

Deuteronomy 33:26-28

26 "There is none like unto the God of Jeshurun, who rideth upon the heaven in thy help, and in his excellency on the sky.

27 The eternal God is thy refuge, and underneath are the everlasting arms: and he shall thrust out the enemy from before thee; and shall say, Destroy them.

28 Israel then shall dwell in safety alone: the fountain of Jacob shall be upon a land of corn and wine; also, his heavens shall drop down dew."

Israel will live in safety alone. (Galatians 6:16; Psalms 91:1-16).

Mark 4:35-38

35 "And the same day, when the even was come, he saith unto them, let us pass over unto the other side.

36 And when they had sent away the multitude, they took him even as he was in the ship. And there were also with him other little ships.

37 And there arose a great storm of wind, and the waves beat into the ship, so that it was now full.

38 And he was in the hinder part of the ship, asleep on a pillow: and they awake him, and say unto him, Master, carest thou not that we perish?"

Jesus was asleep in a stormy boat at sea.

Jonah 1:1-6

1 "Now the word of the LORD came unto Jonah the son of Amittai, saying,

2 Arise, go to Nineveh, that great city, and cry against it; for their wickedness is come up before me.

3 But Jonah rose up to flee unto Tarshish from the presence of the LORD, and went down to Joppa; and he found a ship going to Tarshish: so, he paid the fare thereof, and went down into it, to go with them unto Tarshish from the presence of the LORD.

4 But the LORD sent out a great wind into the sea, and there was a mighty tempest in the sea, so that the ship was like to be broken.

5 Then the mariners were afraid, and cried every man unto his

god, and cast forth the wares that were in the ship into the sea, to lighten it of them. But Jonah was gone down into the sides of the ship; and he lay, and was fast asleep.

6 So the shipmaster came to him, and said unto him, what meanest thou, O sleeper? arise, call upon thy God, if so, be that God will think upon us, that we perish not."

Jonah slept a deep sleep in a stormy ship and sea.

"He giveth His beloved sleep". You must be His beloved to be given.

God gives us sound sleep to keep us healthy and fit and sound/whole and preserved blameless spirit, and soul and body.

Stop whatsoever is robbing them of sleep and restore them.

CHAPTER 8

*HELPERS AND GUIDES ALONG
THE WAY TO THE TOP*

Helpers and guides enable us to tap hidden resources in one so that one could do what He was ready to do and created to do.

Miracle workers of the world always do serve as Helpers and Guides to someone. They restore faith in us to feed the 5000 and raise the dead.

Helpers and guides help us walk on water because they make us forget that we do not know how.

A woman, Elizabeth O'Connor at 53 couldn't start dream career.

Why? Because she lacked the know-how. Then she met a man Mr. Lou O, a specialist in her chosen career who offered her a 3-year course running once a week. Because of the time, cost and her current engagements, she couldn't go at 57 years, the burden had not lifted. So, she went back to Lou. "Am I too old?" she asked Lou.

"Forget about age," Lou said. "There are people who are old at 25 and people who are young at 85. Never let age be a deterrent."

Then he added, "I do have a new requirement since you were here last. I will accept you into my programme only after you have begun work with 2 groups in Washington and are meeting weekly with the group consultant to whom I will refer you."

"How can I manage that?" she responded in utter disbelief.

"Have no fear," Lou said. "You will do it."

Elizabeth O'connor said, "His words were both supporting and challenging, a programme that would have seemed out of my reach up until that moment filled me with the kind of exhilaration, the mountain climbers must know as he sets out to climb his highest peak."

Helpers and Guides along the way tell us, "you will do it." Then encourage, challenge and motivate us. They bring out the best buried in us. They show us that all our challenges are nothing and cannot stop us only if we want to move ahead and rise up to the top. They show us that age or all of our excuses are not sufficient facts to stop us. They make us move ahead until we arrive our destiny. Helpers and Guides provide supernatural aid whenever we need it.

Please listen to me; you will do it. There is nothing confronting you now as a challenge that is meant to stop you.

Is it past failures? Is it lack of enough education? Is it lack of capital? Is it lack of idea? Whatever it is, you name it, cannot hinder it. You can do it and you will do it. All you need is go back to Helpers and Guides on the way.

They Are there in form of Living Books inspired by The Holy Spirit.

Above all, The Holy Spirit is sent as our Help, Guide, Counselor or Comforter.

You need him. As the father now in the Name of Jesus and He will give you The Holy Spirit (Luke 11:13). The Holy Spirit's presence ends all your life's frustrations.

John 14:26

"But the Comforter, which is the Holy Ghost, whom the Father will send in my name, he shall teach you all things, and bring all things to your remembrance, whatsoever I have said unto you."

John 15:26

"But when the Comforter is come, whom I will send unto you from the Father, even the Spirit of truth, which proceeds from the

Father, he shall testify of me:"

John 16:7,13-15

7 "Nevertheless I tell you the truth; It is expedient for you that I go away: for if I go not away, the Comforter will not come unto you; but if I depart, I will send him unto you.

13 Howbeit when he, the Spirit of truth, is come, he will guide you into all truth: for he shall not speak of himself; but whatsoever he shall hear, that shall he speak: and he will shew you things to come.

14 He shall glorify me: for he shall receive of mine, and shall shew it unto you.

15 All things that the Father hath are mine: therefore said I, that he shall take of mine, and shall shew it unto you."

1John 2:20,27

20 "But ye have an unction from the Holy One, and ye know all things.

27 But the anointing which ye have received of him abideth in you, and ye need not that any man teach you: but as the same anointing teacheth you of all things, and is truth, and is no lie, and even as it hath taught you, ye shall abide in him."

Zechariah 4:6

"Then he answered and spake unto me, saying, this is the word of the LORD unto Zerubbabel, saying, Not by might, nor by power, but by my spirit, saith the LORD of hosts."

Isaiah 11:2

"And the spirit of the LORD shall rest upon him, the spirit of wisdom and understanding, the spirit of counsel and might, the spirit of knowledge and of the fear of the LORD;"

CHAPTER 9

WHY YOU CANNOT AND MUST NOT BE SICK

John 15:1-8

1 "I am the true vine, and my Father is the husbandman.

2 Every branch in me that beareth not fruit he taketh away: and every branch that beareth fruit, he purges it, that it may bring forth more fruit.

3 Now ye are clean through the word which I have spoken unto you.

4 Abide in me, and I in you. As the branch cannot bear fruit of itself, except it abide in the vine; no more can ye, except ye abide in me.

5 I am the vine, ye are the branches: He that abideth in me, and I in him, the same bringeth forth much fruit: for without me ye can do nothing.

6 If a man abide not in me, he is cast forth as a branch, and is withered; and men gather them, and cast them into the fire, and they are burned.

7 If ye abide in me, and my words abide in you, ye shall ask what ye will, and it shall be done unto you.

8 Herein is my Father glorified, that ye bear much fruit; so, shall ye be my disciples."

It is God's Glory that you bear much fruit.

God is the Best and Greatest Farmer.

Genesis 2:8

"And the LORD God planted a garden eastward in Eden; and there he put the man whom he had formed."

John 15:1ff.

There is no cocoa farmer that desires fruit from his coca plant/tree that watches pests/insects to destroy his coca plant. Once anything that is hazardous to the life and health of the tree is noticed, it is treated and dealt with immediately so that the tree will keep bearing fruits.

You are a branch of God, most productive tree/plant- the vine. Without your health established, your fruit is worthless.

God treats (personally, by Himself) all branches of His tree that is producing fruit. (John 15:1-4).

God eradicates all forms of disease, sickness, illness, etc from the lives of His chosen ones that are committed to serving Him faithfully by bearing fruits- Growing out what He gives to them.

The best way to remain free from sickness/disease is to be devotedly dedicated to a life time of absolute service to the LORD.

There is NOTHING He cannot do to keep you healthy.

The secrete to the healthy life is service- absolute dedicated service to God on a daily basis. This is the key.

Manage your mind. Whatever happens there will happen in your life in time!

YOUTHS BEWARE! OF SMOKING WEED- (INDIAN HEMP)

Smoking weed is the surest way to weed yourself out of your glorious destiny.

Weed is not what God gave to man as a means to power and rulership. The SEED is it. Never the weed. Why not embrace the seed today for the weed.

Whereas the weed destroys, ruins, and leads to slavery, the seed builds, empowers and leads to your dominion over all things. Go for the seed and not the weed.

The weed is for the weak. The seed is for the strong. The weed is for those who have got no liver. The seed is for all who know what is right. The weed is for the timed, little years.

is right. The weed is for the timed, little years.

CHAPTER 10

ETERNALLY SICKNESS FREE

Proverbs 4:22- They (God's Living Words) are life unto those that FIND THEM. AND HEALTH TO ALL THEIR FLESH.

The Living Word must be searched if one expects to FIND THEM.

But once FOUND, they are LIFE and HEALTH to ALL THEIR FLESH.

Health is the opposite of sickness/disease.

To be healthy is to be sick free and disease free.

Life is the absence of death.

To have health in ALL YOUR FLESH- your whole physical body simply put means that THERE (WOULD BE/IS) NO ROOM FOR SICKNESS/DISEASE IN ANY PART OF YOUR BODY.

Conditions for taking the medication

1.Attend-Give undivided attention, concentration.

2.Incline thine Ear. Be humble and teachable. Take away all prejudices.

3.Let The Living Word never depart from thine Eyes- stay focused on God's words, meditate on The Living Word always.

4.Keep The Living Word in the midst of thine heart- meditate on The Living Word in your heart. (Proverbs 4:23).

The fulfillment of God's Living Word doesn't depend on external circumstances and conditions no matter how negative or adverse it may seem or be.

Logos- The Word of God.

Rhema- Discovered word of God for personal application. It is seen/discovered truth from the living word of God.

You must hear it and it comes alive in you to meet your need.

Philippians 4:19

"But my God shall supply all your need according to his riches in glory by Christ Jesus."

Psalms 23:1

"The LORD is my shepherd; I shall not want."

Psalms 34:10

"The young lions do lack, and suffer hunger: but they that seek the LORD shall not want any good thing."

Psalms 84:11

"For the LORD God is a sun and shield: the LORD will give grace and glory: no good thing will he withhold from them that walk uprightly."

Psalms 118:25

"Save now, I beseech thee, O LORD: O LORD, I beseech thee, send now prosperity."

Dereck Prince took the medicine thrice daily after his meals during world war 11 after he had been sick and had been in the hospital for 12 months without improvement. It was in Egypt. The heat of the sun aggravated his sick condition. Doctors are helpless. They had not the means to neither heal him nor help him. He turned over to The Living Word. Abandoned all his medications for The Living Word. He contacted Romans 10:17 and Proverbs 4:20-22 and took The Living Word as his medication. Within 3 months, he was perfectly healed although he was transferred to Sudan where the condition was worst. Others were feeling critically ill. But he got healed and remained supernaturally healthy.

Hear his own statement- "I made contact with a source of life above the natural levels which is still at work in my physical body today-35yrs have passed since then. That was in 1977. He was born on 14-08-1915 and died on 24-09-2003 at 88 years free from sickness for 72years.

Balm of Gilead.

Jeremiah 8:18-22

18 "When I would comfort myself against sorrow, my heart is faint in me. 19 Behold the voice of the cry of the daughter of my people because of them that dwell in a far country: Is not the LORD in Zion? is not her king in her? Why have they provoked me to anger with their graven images, and with strange vanities?

20 The harvest is past, the summer is ended, and we are not saved.

21 For the hurt of the daughter of my people am I hurt; I am black; astonishment hath taken hold on me.

22 Is there no balm in Gilead; is there no physician there? why then is not the health of the daughter of my people recovered?"

Jeremiah 46:11

"Go up into Gilead, and take balm, O virgin, the daughter of Egypt: in vain shalt thou use many medicines; for thou shalt not be cured."

Restore Healing/Health.

Jeremiah 30:13,17

13 "There is none to plead thy cause, that thou mayest be bound up: thou hast no healing medicines.

17 For I will restore health unto thee, and I will heal thee of thy wounds, saith the LORD; because they called thee an Outcast, saying, This is Zion, whom no man seeks after."

Jeremiah 33:6-12

6 "Behold, I will bring it health and cure, and I will cure them, and will reveal unto them the abundance of peace and truth.

7 And I will cause the captivity of Judah and the captivity of Israel to return, and will build them, as at the first.

8 And I will cleanse them from all their iniquity, whereby they have sinned against me; and I will pardon all their iniquities, whereby they have sinned, and whereby they have transgressed against me.

9 And it shall be to me a name of joy, a praise and an honour be-

fore all the nations of the earth, which shall hear all the good that I do unto them: and they shall fear and tremble for all the goodness and for all the prosperity that I procure unto it.

10 Thus saith the LORD; Again, there shall be heard in this place, which ye say shall be desolate without man and without beast, even in the cities of Judah, and in the streets of Jerusalem, that are desolate, without man, and without inhabitant, and without beast,

11 The voice of joy, and the voice of gladness, the voice of the bridegroom, and the voice of the bride, the voice of them that shall say, Praise the LORD of hosts: for the LORD is good; for his mercy endures forever: and of them that shall bring the sacrifice of praise into the house of the LORD. For I will cause to return the captivity of the land, as at the first, saith the LORD.

12 Thus saith the LORD of hosts; Again, in this place, which is desolate without man and without beast, and in all the cities thereof, shall be a habitation of shepherds causing their flocks to lie down."

Give Health/Cure and cleansing and Salvation and deliverance, fortification/Establishment, Goodness and Prosperity. The voices of Joy, gladness, bridegroom, bride, of all that say praise the Lord of Hosts.

Christ's Ambassadors Living Mission (CALM)

Jeremiah 42:1,10

1 "Then all the captains of the forces, and Johanan the son of Kareah, and Jezaniah the son of Hoshaiah, and all the people from the least even unto the greatest, came near,

10 If ye will still abide in this land, then will I build you, and not pull you down, and I will plant you, and not pluck you up: for I repent me of the evil that I have done unto you."

All the people from the least to the greatest came near to hear and receive The Lord's Instruction. Hear what the Lord God says: "If ye still abide in this land (CALM) then will I build you. And I will plant you. Only the Raised-up ones will be Built and Planted.

RAISE, BUILD AND PLANT/ESTABLISH ALL from the LEAST TO THE GREATEST; All the Captains of the forces and all the people.

Jeremiah 46:27B

... "for, behold, I will save thee from afar off, and thy seed from the land of their captivity; and Jacob shall return, and be in rest and at ease, and none shall make him afraid."

Complete and Total Restoration for all in CALM. Amen!

Jeremiah 50:5,33-34

5 "They shall ask the way to Zion with their faces thitherward, saying, Come, and let us join ourselves to the LORD in a perpetual covenant that shall not be forgotten.

33 Thus saith the LORD of hosts; The children of Israel and the children of Judah were oppressed together: and all that took them captives held them fast; they refused to let them go.

34 Their Redeemer is strong; the LORD of hosts is his name: he shall thoroughly plead their cause, that he may give rest to the land, and disquiet the inhabitants of Babylon."

Jeremiah 50:6-7

6 "My people hath been lost sheep: their shepherds have caused them to go astray, they have turned them away on the mountains: they have gone from mountain to hill, they have forgotten their resting-place.

7 All that found them have devoured them: and their adversaries said, we offend not, because they have sinned against the LORD, the habitation of justice, even the LORD, the hope of their fathers."

CALMERS BEWARE. Take care of the flock.

Jeremiah 50:15

"Shout against her round about: she hath given her hand: her foundations are fallen, her walls are thrown down: for it is the vengeance of the LORD: take vengeance upon her; as she hath done, do unto her."

Destroy the foundation and destroy the structure.

The Living Word sent to destroy all enemies migrating into God's Reserved tree/land.

Jeremiah 47:6-7

6 "O thou sword of the LORD, how long will it be ere thou be quiet? put up thyself into thy scabbard, rest, and be still.

7 How can it be quiet, seeing the LORD hath given it a charge against Ashkelon, and against the sea shore? there hath he appointed it."

Jeremiah 50:21-26,35-37

21 "Go up against the land of Merathaim, even against it, and against the inhabitants of Pekod: waste and utterly destroy after them, saith the LORD, and do according to all that I have commanded thee.

22 A sound of battle is in the land, and of great destruction.

23 How is the hammer of the whole earth cut asunder and broken! how is Babylon become a desolation among the nations!

24 I have laid a snare for thee, and thou art also taken, O Babylon, and thou wast not aware: thou art found, and also caught, because thou hast striven against the LORD.

25 The LORD hath opened his armoury, and hath brought forth the weapons of his indignation: for this is the work of the Lord GOD of hosts in the land of the Chaldeans.

26 Come against her from the utmost border, open her storehouses: cast her up as heaps, and destroy her utterly: let nothing of her be left.

35 A sword is upon the Chaldeans, saith the LORD, and upon the inhabitants of Babylon, and upon her princes, and upon her wise men.

36 A sword is upon the liars; and they shall dote: a sword is upon her mighty men; and they shall be dismayed.

37 A sword is upon their horses, and upon their chariots, and upon all the mingled people that are in the midst of her; and they shall become as women: a sword is upon her treasures; and they shall be robbed."

Jeremiah 51:1-3

1 "Thus saith the LORD; Behold, I will raise up against Babylon, and against them that dwell in the midst of them that rise up against me, a destroying wind;

2 And will send unto Babylon fanners, that shall fan her, and shall empty her land: for in the day of trouble they shall be against her round about.

3 Against him that bends let the archer bend his bow, and against him that lifts himself up in his brigandine: and spare ye not her young men; destroy ye utterly all her host."

CALMERS ARE FANNERS.

Jeremiah 51:1-2

1 "Thus saith the LORD; Behold, I will raise up against Babylon, and against them that dwell in the midst of them that rise up against me, a destroying wind;

2 And will send unto Babylon fanners, that shall fan her, and shall empty her land: for in the day of trouble they shall be against her round about."

CALM IS ZION. Jeremiah 51:5-6, 8B,10, 15-23,29-30,45.

Healing in CALM/ZION.

Lamentation 2:3

"He hath cut off in his fierce anger all the horn of Israel: he hath drawn back his right hand from before the enemy, and he burned against Jacob like a flaming fire, which devours round about."

Jeremiah 8:19-22

19 "Behold the voice of the cry of the daughter of my people because of them that dwell in a far country: Is not the LORD in Zion? is not her king in her? Why have they provoked me to anger with their graven images, and with strange vanities?

20 The harvest is past, the summer is ended, and we are not saved."

Jeremiah 46:11

Go up into Gilead, and take balm, O virgin, the daughter of Egypt: in vain shalt thou use many medicines; for thou shalt not be cured.

Jeremiah 51:8b,10

Verse 8b of Jeremiah 51 says "howl for her; take balm for her pain, if so, be she may be healed.

10 The LORD hath brought forth our righteousness: come, and let us declare in Zion the work of the LORD our God."

Proverbs 4:20-22- The Living Word is life and Health to All our Flesh.

- Attend

- Incline thine Ear unto my words.
- Keep them in the midst of thine Eyes.
- Keep them in the midst of thine heart.

55

CHAPTER 11

SET ALL FREE FROM SIN AND SICKNESS

Set all free from sin and sickness and they will be freed from poverty!

Believers are struggling with sin and sickness today more than ever before.

And whoever struggles with sin and sickness will most assuredly, unfailingly struggle/better still live with poverty.

Until the sin and sickness problems are dealt with, the enemy won't stop ravaging the church with poverty.

Sin brings poverty to the believer whether he likes it or not. Genesis 3:23-24.

Sickness forces him into poverty even against his/her will- Mark 5:25-26.

For this purpose, Jesus came-1John 3:8.

He bore sins.

Isaiah 53:3-5

3 "He is despised and rejected of men; a man of sorrows, and acquainted with grief: and we hid as it were our faces from him; he was despised, and we esteemed him not. {we hid...: or, he hid as it were his face from us: Heb. as a hiding of faces from him, or, from us}

4 Surely, he hath borne our griefs, and carried our sorrows: yet

we did esteem him stricken, smitten of God, and afflicted.

5 But he was wounded for our transgressions, he was bruised for our iniquities: the chastisement of our peace was upon him; and with his stripes we are healed."

1Peter 2:24.

"Who his own self bare our sins in his own body on the tree, that we, being dead to sins, should live unto righteousness: by whose stripes ye were healed."

He carried our sicknesses.

Isaiah 53:3-5

3 "He is despised and rejected of men; a man of sorrows, and acquainted with grief: and we hid as it were our faces from him; he was despised, and we esteemed him not. {we hid...: or, he hid as it were his face from us: Heb. as a hiding of faces from him, or, from us}

4 Surely, he hath borne our griefs, and carried our sorrows: yet we did esteem him stricken, smitten of God, and afflicted.

5 But he was wounded for our transgressions, he was bruised for our iniquities: the chastisement of our peace was upon him; and with his stripes we are healed."

Matthew 8:17

"That it might be fulfilled which was spoken by Esaias the prophet, saying, Himself took our infirmities, and bare our sicknesses."

He was made sin, sick, and poor for my sake.

1Peter 2:24.

"Who his own self bare our sins in his own body on the tree, that we, being dead to sins, should live unto righteousness: by whose stripes ye were healed."

Isaiah 53:3-5

3 "He is despised and rejected of men; a man of sorrows, and acquainted with grief: and we hid as it were our faces from him; he was despised, and we esteemed him not. {we hid...: or, he hid as it were his face from us: Heb. as a hiding of faces from him, or, from us}

4 Surely, he hath borne our griefs, and carried our sorrows: yet

we did esteem him stricken, smitten of God, and afflicted.

5 But he was wounded for our transgressions, he was bruised for our iniquities: the chastisement of our peace was upon him; and with his stripes we are healed."

2Corinthians 8:9

"For ye know the grace of our Lord Jesus Christ, that, though he was rich, yet for your sakes he became poor, that ye through his poverty might be rich."

There is no justifiable reason today why I should suffer carrying what Jesus bore and took away. That is Ridiculous.

If we (CAMBS) succeed in freeing mankind from sin and sickness via the gospel, we will enrich them with prosperity- Luke 4:18-19; Isaiah 61:1-4.

Most believers who think sin must not be mentioned or associated with them, very gladly welcomes sickness/disease/illness with their whole heart.

What a Christian we are!

The same price Jesus paid, at the same time, via His Blood settled all the problems of sin, sickness and poverty.

We are not experiencing any of these evil vices Satan brought to man after all Jesus had done for us. Disease/sickness is not an expression of love and so doesn't come from God the Father who is love and gives good gift-James 1:17.

I cannot sin because I have His seed in me.

I cannot be sick because I have his life/health.

I cannot be poor because I have His prosperity.

What Jesus did settle once and for all everything that Satan did, is doing and will ever do to affect me negatively.

If it is wrong for me to pay for my sin/bear them, it is similarly very wrong for me to bear any sickness, disease or illness/curses/ poverty after Jesus bore them all in my stead/behalf.

It is the Father's will that we be as free from sickness as we are of sin.

Spiritual death gave birth to physical death. In likewise manner, spiritual life gives birth to physical life, health, soundness, wellbeing and wholeness.

John 10:10

"The thief cometh not, but for to steal, and to kill, and to destroy: I am come that they might have life, and that they might have it more abundantly."

When Jesus came into our hearts, He brought in life and immortality-Romans 1:16; 2Timothy 1:10; 2Corinthians 4:10-11B.

If the spiritual death of Adam gave birth to physical death of man, then more so will the spiritual/eternal life of Christ give birth to my total soundness and health-see 1Corinthians 15:45-49.

Hebrews 7:22

"By so much was Jesus made a surety of a better testament."

Jesus is the surety of the New Covenant.

Hebrews 9:26

"For then must he often have suffered since the foundation of the world: but now once in the end of the world hath he appeared to put away sin by the sacrifice of himself."

Once at the end of the ages, Jesus was manifested to put away sin by the sacrifice of Himself.

Note: When He put sin away, all after math of sin-poverty, sickness, disease, curses, etc were equally put away.

He carried them away-Matthew 8:17; Hebrews 9:26; and we have no reason, legally, morally, logically whatsoever to bring back what Jesus carried away. Halleluyah!

Hebrews 10:12

"But this man, after he had offered one sacrifice for sins forever, sat down on the right hand of God;"

Jesus offered one sacrifice forever for sin, sickness, poverty, etc.

Why must any saved child of God allow the devil put on him/her what Jesus hath fully paid for-once and for all.

If Jesus sacrifice for our sins didn't make us better than Adam before his fall, then God failed in His Redemptive plan.

The plan of God was to Recover man and Preserve him blameless so that He cannot fall like Adam anymore.

Psalms 121:6-8

6 "The sun shall not smite thee by day, nor the moon by night.

7 The LORD shall preserve thee from all evil: he shall preserve thy soul.

8 The LORD shall preserve thy going out and thy coming in from this time forth, and even for evermore."

1 Thessalonians 5:23-24

24 "Faithful is he that calleth you, who also will do it.

25 Brethren, pray for us."

1John 2:1-3.

1 "My little children, these things write I unto you, that ye sin not. And if any man sin, we have an advocate with the Father, Jesus Christ the righteous:

2 And he is the propitiation for our sins: and not for ours only, but also for the sins of the whole world.

3 And hereby we do know that we know him, if we keep his commandments."

2Corinthians 4:10-11

10 "Always bearing about in the body the dying of the Lord Jesus, that the life also of Jesus might be made manifest in our body.

11 For we which live are always delivered unto death for Jesus' sake, that the life also of Jesus might be made manifest in our mortal flesh."

2Corinthians 5:4-5

4 "For we that are in this tabernacle do groan, being burdened: not for that we would be unclothed, but clothed upon, that mortality might be swallowed up of life.

5 Now he that hath wrought us for the selfsame thing is God, who also hath given unto us the earnest of the Spirit."

Our mortal body is to be swallowed up of life when we receive the gospel.

Romans 1:16

"For I am not ashamed of the gospel of Christ: for it is the power of God unto salvation to everyone that believeth; to the Jew first, and also to the Greek."

2Timothy 1:10

"But is now made manifest by the appearing of our Saviour

Jesus Christ, who hath abolished death, and hath brought life and immortality to light through the gospel:"

That means every trace of sickness and disease is to be swallowed up by the life of Christ in you the same way Moses rod swallowed the rods of the Egyptians. (See Exodus 7:10-12).

Mortality implies weakness, sickness, death.

Immortality implies divine strength, divine health and eternal or divine life.

Jesus Christ has brought to us God's own very kind of life as He has it now. That is what immortality connotes: God's very life in the body of man swallowing up everything in man that makes man mortal and transplanting everything that makes God immortal into man to transform and translate man into immortality. This is what the Gospel is all about: To make man exactly like God by making him like Christ who is God made flesh.

The life of Jesus is to be manifested in our mortal flesh bringing about solid, unstained health. This is total preservation from sickness, disease, illness, evils and every trace of wickedness. This is the very plan and purpose of God that Jesus Christ came to enforce for mankind. And this is the very reason why The Lord Jesus Christ sent me as His Ambassador: To restore this divine life and health to all who will believe.

Remember what The Holy Spirit said to me as documented in the First Words!

To be Healed, you do nothing!

You are not to labour to be Healed You are not to wear yourself out in search of healing or spend fortunes to secure healing. You merely look put The Lord or come by faith to receive what belongs to you and has been fully paid for.

God says "Himself [Jesus Christ] bore our sins in His own body on the tree, that we, having died to sins, might live for righteousness--by whose stripes you were healed." 1Peter 2:24

Notice what God says: By whose stripes you were healed! If 'YOU were healed' then 'YOU are healed'!

"He [Jesus Christ] Himself took our infirmities [or diseases] and bore our sicknesses." Matthew 8:17

Notice again what God who cannot lie says about you: Himself [Jesus Christ] TOOK YOUR diseases and BORE [carried away] YOUR sicknesses. What Jesus Christ took and carried away and destroyed on the TREE where He was crucified and declared IT IS FINISHED stands finished forever! That settles the problem of sickness and disease forever for all who will believe! All you need to do is to believe and receive!

Jesus Christ speaking in John 3:14-17 says "And as Moses lifted up the serpent in the wilderness, even so must the Son of man be lifted up: That whosoever believeth in him should not perish, but have eternal life. For God so loved the world, that he gave his only begotten Son, that whosoever believeth in him should not perish, but have everlasting life. For God sent not his Son into the world to condemn the world; but that the world through him might be saved [healed, delivered, made whole, restored to sound health and preserved]."

Notice that every single person that was bitten by the serpent in Numbers 21:4-9 that LOOKED on God's provision by faith, LIVED! They didn't do anything to be healed. They only looked and got healed. Whatever was the distance between where they were and where the serpent of brass made by Moses at God's command was placed was immaterial. All that looked by faith got healed instantly and lived. That's how simple healing is for all who will believe in God's Provision today! God never made healing difficult, only religion does.

The Lord God wants all the sick to be healed by faith. LOOK and be healed of any and every sickness.

Healing has never been made simpler! Look up by faith and see Jesus on the Cross and be healed and live.

This Book is on a Divine Assignment and Mission: To Bring to YOU all The Living Word made flesh brought to the people of God in His days on earth. Read with an open heart. Its YOUR season of Restoration to God's Divine Health Plan. You shall not die sick but be healed and live. And all you need now is Faith! Only believe and YOU will see the salvation, healing, restoration and glory of the Lord.

Believe and Look up to The Lord of Glory and Live.

I decree your total healing from the crown of your head to the soles of your feet in Jesus Name.

I proclaim your Liberty and Restoration to All Jesus paid and owns now in Jesus Name.

Peace in Jesus Precious Name!

I am expecting your testimonies.

BECOME A CITIZEN OF HEAVEN TODAY!

Please note, if you are not yet a Citizen of Heaven, but desire to be, this is your opportunity. To be a citizen of Heaven, you must be from above. You must be born of God. You must be born again!

John 3:3-8,12-13

3 Jesus answered and said to him, "Most assuredly, I say to you, unless one is born again, he cannot see the kingdom of God."

4 Nicodemus said to Him, "How can a man be born when he is old? Can he enter a second time into his mother's womb and be born?"

5 Jesus answered, "Most assuredly, I say to you, unless one is born of water and the Spirit, he cannot enter the kingdom of God.

6 "That which is born of the flesh is flesh, and that which is born of the Spirit is spirit.

7 "Do not marvel that I said to you, 'You must be born again.'

8 "The wind blows where it wishes, and you hear the sound of it, but cannot tell where it comes from and where it goes. So is everyone who is born of the Spirit."

12 If I have told you earthly things, and ye believe not, how shall ye believe, if I tell you of heavenly things?

13 And no man hath ascended up to heaven, but he that came down from heaven, even the Son of man which is in heaven.

Jesus says "You must be born again to live and enjoy Heaven-now!" John 3:3,7

No matter your sin(s) and what you may have done, God wants you forgive and restored now!

John 3:13-18

13 "No one has ascended to heaven but He who came down from heaven, that is, the Son of Man who is in heaven.

14 "And as Moses lifted up the serpent in the wilderness, even so must the Son of Man be lifted up,

15 "that whoever believes in Him should not perish but have eternal life.

16 "For God so loved the world that He gave His only begotten Son, that whoever believes in Him should not perish but have everlasting life.

17 "For God did not send His Son into the world to condemn the world, but that the world through Him might be saved.

18 "He who believes in Him is not condemned; but he who does not believe is condemned already, because he has not believed in the name of the only begotten Son of God.

Remember God gives the power to become His son to everyone that receives Jesus as The Christ, The Son of The Living God or believe in His Name. John 1:12

Remember God Himself dwells in everyone who believes and confesses that Jesus is The Christ, The Son of The Living God. 1John 5:1, 4-5;1John 4:4,15

Remember God did not send His Son into the world to condemn the world but that through Him, the world might be saved. John 3:17

Beloved, AS the Father sent Jesus The Christ, even so has The Lord Jesus Christ sent me so that everyone who will believe and receive me as His Ambassador will be saved, healed, delivered and restored. The Lord said to me: As the Father sent Me, even so have I sent you! John 17:18; John 20:21

The Lord said to Me: Verily, verily I say to you, whoever receives you receives me, and whoever receives me receives the Father who sent me. John 13:20.

The Lord said to Me: Whoever rejects you rejects me, and whoever rejects Me rejects The Father who sent Me. Luke 10:16

The Lord said to Me: Behold I give unto you power to tread upon serpents and scorpions and over all the power of the enemy and nothing shall by any means hurt you. Luke 10:19

The Lord said to Me: Behold, I send in the midst of many peoples, like dew from the LORD, like showers on the grass, that tarry for no man nor wait for the sons of men. Behold, you shall be among the Gentiles, In the midst of many peoples, like a lion among the beasts of the forest, like a young lion among flocks of sheep, Who, if he passes through, both treads down and tears in pieces, and none can deliver. Your hand shall be lifted against your adversaries, and all your enemies shall be cut off. Micah 5:7-9

The Lord said to Me: You will be like the dew to all My people and creation; You shall grow like the lily, and lengthen Your roots like Lebanon. Your branches shall spread; Your beauty shall be like an olive tree, And Your fragrance like Lebanon. Those who dwell under Your shadow shall return; They shall be revived like grain, and grow like a vine. Their scent shall be like the wine of Lebanon. Hosea 14:5-7

Beloved, there is no justifiable reason under Heaven why you should ever go through ANYTHING that is not in Heaven now!

Beloved there is no justifiable reason why you should not have NOW the best God has fully paid for and credited to your personal account!

Hear Me: All things are ready. And all things are yours! What are you still waiting for? All you need to do is to believe that Jesus is the Christ, The Son of The Living God. And He sent Me to bring this Goodnews to you.

Your struggles can come to an end today. You can be enrolled into Heaven's citizenship right now. You can begin a new life today and enjoy all that is available in Heaven from this day forward. The Lord Jesus Christ who sent me confirms with undeniable proof that He is ALIVE today in the lives of those who hear my words and believes in Him [The Lord Jesus Christ] who sent me.

Jesus is alive today and the only way to prove it is for Him to do what He did before in your life today. He sent me and will prove to you that this is not a made-up story written to impress you, but His ordained will made available to make you are created to be!

The choice is yours! Rise and take what belong to you and enter your rest!

Peace now and always in Jesus Almighty Name!

Amen!!!

If You are not certain that You are Born Again as you are certain of your name, or You were once saved but went astray again, living and doing as you pleased, then say this Prayer aloud now for you to become a citizen of Heaven:

PRAYER FOR SALVATION AND RESTORATION TO HEAVEN'S CITIZENSHIP!

Dear Heavenly Father, I return to you by Faith. I am sorry for my sins. I believe in my heart that Jesus is The Christ and that He died for my sins and rose from the dead on the third day, according to Scripture, for my justification. I confess that Jesus Christ is LORD and I accept Him now as my Saviour. I believe my sins are wiped away.

I call upon The Name of The LORD for my total Healing, Liberty and Restoration.

I ask for the Gift of Your Holy Spirit, Power and Grace to follow and serve You from this day forward. And I Thank You Abba Father for doing far beyond all I have asked and can ever imagine in Jesus Name. Amen!

I Now Declare That I Am A Child of God Forever! There's no going back.

Now that you have become a Citizen of Heaven, you need to upgrade by signing up to serve as an Ambassador for Christ. That is where your security and relevance lie. There is no job in this world that can be compared to serving as The Ambassador of The King of kings and Lord of lords. The benefits are amazing. You cannot do a better or more honourable job.

You can Enlist now and become a Partner or a Member of our Totally Empowered Ambassadors on Mission (TEAM) and see what Our Risen Lord and King Jesus Christ will transform your life into and do in, for and through you from this day as you believe and obey His Word!

I can't wait to hear from you because I believe you have been blessed and helped immensely reading this Book as much as I am writing it! I am praying for you.

ABOUT THE AUTHOR

Amb. Promise Ogbonna

Amb Promise Ogbonna is the President of Christ's Ambassadors Living Mission International Inc. aka Jesus Mission Headquarters, an all-encompassing network of ministries with a mandate focus to Preach The Everlasting Gospel to all, Stop anything after man's destruction, Bring Healing, Liberty and Restoration to all, Make ALL Christ's Ambassadors and Make Heaven-Now a Reality for All.

He is the Publisher of ONTOP Life Publishers Company with a commission to Publish the Everlasting Gospel and Bring God's Wisdom-solutions for every problem and need of mankind.

He represents The Lord Jesus Christ and serves Him as His Ambassador!

He is married and blessed with children.

OTHER BOOKS BY AMB PROMISE OGBONNA

1. The Nothingness of Satan
2. You Can Make a Fresh Start and Rule Your World
3. Restoring The Forgotten Dignity of Woman
4. Christ's Ambassadors: Re-Emergence of Rulers in
5. Why Prophet Elisha Died Sick and how to Avoid it
6. You Can Choose When to Die
7. You Shall Live and Not Die
8. Why Christians Die Sick
9. 7 Keys to Undeniable Healing
10. 8 Decisive Hours That Will Take You To The Topmost
11. Activating God's Medicine For Your Healing
12. God Cannot Fail To Heal You
13. Healing Is Your Legal Right
14. God's Final Solution to The Problem of The Black Race
15. Understanding God's Secret to Winning Life's Battles
16. 100 Years Is Minimum
17. How to Raise The Dead
18. Manifesting ss Signs and Wonders: Unlocking The Unstoppable You Regardless of Where You are Now!
19. 40 Pitfalls to Avoid in Life – Mastering The Art of Living Successfully.
20. Wisdom Seeds to Greatness In Life – Inspiring Seed-Thoughts on Being Your Best
21. God's Medicine for Incurable Diseases
22. Ambassador Promise: Jesus Christ's Official Ambassador and T. L. Osborn's Successor on Earth Today! Appearance and En-

counters with The Lord Jesus Christ, Mantles of Notable Servants of God Received and The 9 Mandates.

UPCOMING BOOKS BY AMB PROMISE OGBONNA

1. Enforcing Kingdom Wealth Transfer
2. God's Final Word on Tithes, Tithing and Offerings
3. Creating Heaven Out of Your Ruined World
4. How to Attract God's Blessing on Your Business and Career
5. How to Make Your Faith Work
6. God's Master Key to Your Dominion
7. Wisdom Keys To God's Recovery Plan
8. Jesus Christ's Teaching on Provoking Our Covenant Heritage of Prosperity
9. Why People Fail in Life –Secrets to Success without Stress

Please visit your favorite eBook retailer to discover other books by Amb Promise Ogbonna.

CONNECT WITH AMB PROMISE OGBONNA

I appreciate you reading my book. Here are my links and Social Coordinates

Send Amb Promise Ogbonna a mail at:

Visit Amb. Promise Ogbonna's Website:

Subscribe to Amb Promise Ogbonna's videos at:

Follow Amb Promise Ogbonna on Twitter:

Friend Amb Promise Ogbonna on Facebook:

Connect with Amb Promise Ogbonna on LinkedIn:

Read Amb Promise Ogbonna's Story at Wattpad:

Subscribe to Amb Promise Ogbonna's Blog at:

Follow Amb Promise Ogbonna on Instagram:

Subscribe to Amb. Promise Ogbonna's HEAVENow You Tube Channel:

Read Amb Promise Ogbonna's Smashwords Interview at

Read Amb Promise Ogbonna's Author Profile at Smashwords:

Follow Amb Promise Ogbonna at Amazon:

Connect with Amb Promise Ogbonna on Pinterest:

Read Amb. Promise Ogbonna books at Okada Books:

Get Access to all the Books of Amb Promise Ogbonna at Books2Read Universal Book Link:

JOIN AMB. PROMISE OGBONNA IN HEAVENOW SERVICES

Worship with Ambassador Promise in Christ's Ambassadors Heaven-Now Services at:

Christ's Ambassadors Living Mission International [Jesus Mission Headquarters]

24 Independence Street, Behind O'Mark Schools by O'Mark Bus Stop, LASU Road, Igando Lagos

Wednesdays: 12:00-1:00pm. Hour of EmPowerment for All [Online]

Saturdays: 8:00-9:00am. Hour of Healing for All

Sundays: 8:00-9:00am. Hour of Liberty and Restoration for All

Sundays: 9:00-10:00am. Hour of Kingdom Wealth Transfer for All

Last Friday Night Monthly: 10pm. Night of Restorations for All

Ambassadors International Bible Institute: Runs Online and Offline Courses to Make Christ's Ambassadors and Make Heaven Now a reality for all. Enroll today!

HEAVENow...Making Heaven now a Reality for ALL!

OUR HEALING PRODUCTS

We are on a Mission to Bring Healing to the sick no matter their sicknesses or diseases and Restore Health, Wealth and Peace to ALL! Here are some of our Products and Services we run to Bring Healing to the sick worldwide!

1. All-Purpose Divine Healing Medicine
2. Healing Messages – Podcasts, CD, MP3 and DVD
3. Healing Books
4. Healing Leaves Magazine
5. Healing Anointing Oil
6. Healing Mantles and Clothes
7. Healing Materials
8. Healing Elixir for incurable diseases
9. Healing Songs
10. Healing Homes
11. Health Centers
12. Healing Balm

Call us today for all of your Healing needs! We are here to SERVE YOU!

OUR SPECIAL SERVICES

We Offer the following services to Churches, Ministries, Corporate Bodies, Businesses, Communities, Groups, International Bodies, NGO's, Governments, States and Nations.

1. Healing Seminars
2. Healing School
3. Healing Teams
4. Healing Outreaches and Explosions
5. World Healing Conferences
6. Health and Wealth Trainings
7. Heaven-Now Campaigns
8. Kingdom Wealth Transfer Seminars
9. God's FASTEST Prosperity Recovery Seminars
10. Heaven's Business School
11. Time and Stress Management Training
12. Leadership Responsibility Development Training

Our Services are geared towards making every person fit spirit, soul and body so that they can be empowered to deliver results competently, effectively and efficiently.

For Bookings Contact us today!

9 781658 224345